A Practical Book of

PHARMACOLOGY - III

As Per PCI Regulations

THIRD YEAR B. PHARM.
Semester - VI

Dr. Manjunatha P. Mudagal

Professor & HOD,
Department of Pharmacology,
Acharya Dr. Sarvepalli Radhakrishna Road
Acharya PO, Soladevanahalli,
Bengaluru-560 107, Karnataka, India

Mr. T. Hari Babu

Assistant Professor
Department of Pharmacology,
Acharya Dr. Sarvepalli Radhakrishna Road
Acharya PO, Soladevanahalli,
Bengaluru-560 107, Karnataka, India

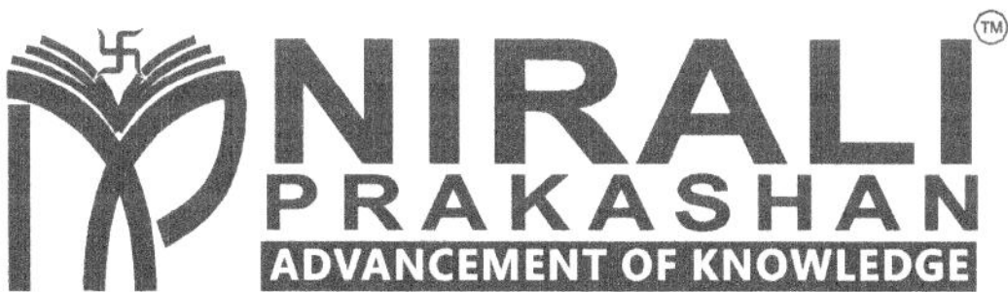

N4093

A Practical Book of Pharmacology - III   **ISBN**

First Edition   : **January 2020**
©   : **Author**

Published By :
NIRALI PRAKASHAN
Abhyudaya Pragati, 1312, Shivaji Nagar,
Off J.M. Road, PUNE – 411005
Tel - (020) 25512336/37/39, Fax - (020) 25511379
Email : niralipune@pragationline.com

☞ DISTRIBUTION CENTRES

PUNE

Nirali Prakashan : 119, Budhwar Peth, Jogeshwari Mandir Lane, Pune 411002, Maharashtra
(For orders within Pune)   Tel : (020) 2445 2044, Fax : (020) 2445 1538; Mobile : 9657703145
Email : bookorder@pragationline.com, niralilocal@pragationline.com

Nirali Prakashan : S. No. 28/27, Dhyari, Near Pari Company, Pune 411041
(For orders outside Pune)   Tel : (020) 24690204 Fax : (020) 24690316; Mobile : 9657703143
Email : dhyari@pragationline.com, bookorder@pragationline.com

MUMBAI

Nirali Prakashan : 385, S.V.P. Road, Rasdhara Co-op. Hsg. Society Ltd.,
Girgaum, Mumbai 400004, Maharashtra; Mobile : 9320129587
Tel : (022) 2385 6339 / 2386 9976, Fax : (022) 2386 9976
Email : niralimumbai@pragationline.com

☞ DISTRIBUTION BRANCHES

JALGAON

Nirali Prakashan : 34, V. V. Golani Market, Navi Peth, Jalgaon 425001,
Maharashtra, Tel : (0257) 222 0395, Mob : 94234 91860

KOLHAPUR

Nirali Prakashan : New Mahadvar Road, Kedar Plaza, 1st Floor Opp. IDBI Bank
Kolhapur 416 012, Maharashtra. Mob : 9850046155

NAGPUR

Nirali Prakashan : Above Maratha Mandir, Shop No. 3, First Floor,
Rani Jhanshi Square, Sitabuldi, Nagpur 440012, Maharashtra
Tel : (0712) 254 7129

DELHI

Nirali Prakashan : 4593/15, Basement, Agarwal Lane, Ansari Road, Daryaganj
Near Times of India Building, New Delhi 110002 Mob : 08505972553
Email : niralidelhi@pragationline.com

BENGALURU

Nirali Prakashan : Maitri Ground Floor, Jaya Apartments, No. 99, 6th Cross, 6th Main,
Malleswaram, Bengaluru 560003, Karnataka; Mob : 9449043034
Email: niralibangalore@pragationline.com

Other Branches : Hyderabad, Chennai

niralipune@pragationline.com　|　www.pragationline.com
Also find us on 🅕 www.facebook.com/niralibooks

Preface

It is our immense pleasure to bring out the "First Edition" of this book which is dedicated to the students and faculty of B. Pharma institutes of this country. This book is designed and edited in accordance to the syllabus requirement of **"Pharmacology-III"** of third year (6th Semester) B. Pharm course in pharmacy prescribed in **"Bachelor of Pharmacy (B. Pharm) course regulations 2014"** by Pharmacy council of India.

Sincere efforts have been made to present experimental details along with pre-experimental aspects viz., vehicle of choice, drug dissolution and volume selection rational, preparation of stock solution and working standards with examples used in experimental pharmacology. Most experiments are described stating examples with an intention to scaffold experimental procedures attempted during Pharmacology Practical sessions to various global organizations.

Core concepts and underlying principles have been discussed for every experiment, making the practical study meaningful and helpful to understand the objective of the experiments. Certain experiments adopted with OECD guidelines, Illustrations with observational values for few experiments, precautions and overcoming errors will act as a pragmatic guideline for the students and make students better understanding with the concepts.

We are thankful to the **management** of **Acharya & BM Reddy College of Pharmacy, Bengaluru** for their keen interest and timely encouragement that made it possible to bring out this first volume.

We are highly indebted to **Dr. Divakar Goli**, professor & Mentor, Acharya & BM Reddy College of Pharmacy, Bengaluru for his constant motivation and guidance.

Suggestions and comments are always welcome and they shall be gratefully acknowledged.

Manjunatha P. Mudagal

T. Hari Babu

Syllabus

1. Dose calculation in pharmacological experiments.

2. Antiallergic activity by mast cell stabilization assay.

3. Study of anti-ulcer activity of a drug using pylorus ligand (SHAY) rat model and NSAIDS induced ulcer model.

4. Study of effect of drugs on gastrointestinal motility.

5. Effect of agonist and antagonists on guinea pig ileum.

6. Estimation of serum biochemical parameters by using semi-autoanalyser.

7. Effect of saline purgative on frog intestine.

8. Insulin hypoglycemic effect in rabbit.

9. Test for pyrogens (rabbit method).

10. Determination of acute oral toxicity (LD50) of a drug from a given data.

11. Determination of acute skin irritation / corrosion of a test substance.

12. Determination of acute eye irritation / corrosion of a test substance.

13. Calculation of pharmacokinetic parameters from a given data.

14. Biostatistics methods in experimental pharmacology (student's t test, ANOVA).

15. Biostatistics methods in experimental pharmacology (Chi square test, Wilcoxon Signed Rank test).

Contents

Experiment No. 01
Dose Calculation in Pharmacological Experiments

Aim: *To calculate dose in Pharmacological Experiments.*

Introduction:

Experimental animals have been of very important tools in the history of non-human research models for scientific purposes in almost every aspect of biomedical, behavioral researches and testing conducted in Colleges, Universities, Medical schools, Pharmaceutical companies, Research institutes, Farms and Commercial facilities that provide animal-testing services to industry. Experiments on animals are necessary in drugs discovery and development as well as to advance medical and biological knowledge. Dosage calculation and stock solution preparation based on dosage rationale formula are prerequisites to drug administration in experimental animals. However, drugs dosage calculations and stock solution preparations are not clearly explained in most scientific literatures involving the use of experimental animals, and this is a major challenge to some undergraduate students, post-graduate students and other researchers. Since over 90% of animals used in *in-vivo* experiments in medical, physiological, pharmacological, chemical, toxicological, biological, biochemical and genetic studies are rats and mice, this work is aimed to simplify calculation of doses, preparation of stock solution in experimental animal for the benefits of all researchers.

(a) Vehicle of choice, drugs dissolution and volume selection rationale:

- A vehicle is any substance that acts as a medium in which a drug is administered.

- Vehicle, which is an essential consideration in all animal research should be biologically inert, have no toxic effects on the animals and not also influence the results obtained for the compound under investigation. Example of suitable vehicles for animal research include; water, normal saline (0.9% sodium chloride), 50% polyethylene glycol, 5 to 10% Tween 80, 0.25% methyl cellulose or carboxy methyl cellulose (CMC).

- In most researches involving experimental animals, dosages are usually calculated from stock solution of the test drugs dissolved in appropriate volume of solvent (vehicle).

- According to the OECD's (Organization of Economic Co-operation and Development) guidelines, dosage of drug (mg) should be constituted in an appropriate volume not usually exceeding 10 ml/kg (1 ml/100 g) body weight of experimental animals (mice and rats) for non-aqueous solvent in oral route of administration.

- In the case of aqueous solvents, 20 ml/kg (2 ml/100 g) body weight can be considered (OECD, 2000).

- Large dose volumes (40 ml/kg body weight) can cause unnecessary stress to animals and can also overload the stomach capacity and pass immediately into the small bowel or can result in passive reflux in the stomach, aspiration pneumonia, pharyngeal, esophageal, and gastric irritation or injury with stricture formation, esophageal and gastric rupture and stress.

- Lower volume (5 ml/kg) can be considered to dissolve highly soluble solute drugs. Such low volume would ease the administration of drug in solution.
- However, highly viscous drug solution should be diluted, whenever possible, for ease of administration. However, final dilution volume should not exceed 20 ml/kg.

OECD's Guideline on Volume Selection :

Table 1

Standard volume	Animal's body weight (g)	Calculated volume (ml) based on animal's body weight
10 ml/kg	100 g	1.00 ml
(Appropriate volume)	150 g	1.50 ml
20 ml/kg	100 g	2.00 ml
(Maximum volume)	150 g	3.00 ml

(b) Dosage calculation and preparation of stock solution of crude plant extract for experimental animals:

Stock solutions and doses of a plant extract (With selected doses, 200 mg/kg and 400 mg/kg) for a rat weighing 120 g be calculated as follows:

Step 1: Dosage calculation

Body weight of animal = 120 g

Dosage in mg = Body weight of animal/1000 g × dose (mg)

Dosage in mg = 120 g/ 1000 g × 200 (mg) = 24 mg.

Step 2: Dissolution of dose in a suitable vehicle for oral administration:

From the OECD's guidelines,

120 g rat requires 24 mg of the crude plant extract which should be constituted is not more than 1.2 ml of normal saline (see table 1 above) according to the OECD guideline.

In a nut shell, 120 g ≡ 24 mg ≡ 1.2 ml of normal saline.

Showing stock solutions from two selected doses of a crude plant extract:

Table 2

Selected dose	Stock solution	Animal's body weight (g)	Calculated dose (mg)	Equivalent dose in ml
Low dose, 200 mg/kg	960 mg/48 ml (20 mg/ml)	100 g	24 mg	1.20 ml
		150 g	30 mg	1.50 ml
High dose, 400 mg/kg	960 mg/24 ml (40 mg/ml)	100 g	48 mg	1.20 ml
		150 g	60 mg	1.50 ml

(c) Direct calculation of animal's dose from human dose:

Key Points in Scaling of Dose:

- Larger animals have lower metabolic rates.
- Physiological process of larger animals is slower.
- Larger animals require smaller drug dose on weight basis.
- Allometry accounts the difference in physiological time among species.
- Do not apply allometric scaling to convert adult doses to kids.

Human equivalent dose calculation based on body surface area*

Table 3

Species	Reference body weight (kg)	Working weight range (kg)	Body surface area (m^2)	To convert dose in mg/kg to dose in mg/m^2, multiply by km	To convert animal dose in mg/kg to HED in mg/kg, either	
					Divide animal dose by	Multiply animal dose by
Human	60	–	1.62	37	–	–
Mouse	0.02	0.011 – 0.034	0.07	3	12.3	0.081
Rat	0.15	0.08 – 0.27	0.025	6	6.2	0.162
Guinea pig	0.40	0.208- 0.700	0.05	8	4.6	0.216
Rabbit	1.8	0.90-3.0	0.15	12	3.1	0.324

*Data obtained from FDA draft guidelines. FDA: Food and Drug Administration, HED: Human equivalent dose.

Conclusion:

- Dose estimation always requires careful consideration about the difference in pharmacokinetics and pharmacodynamics among species.
- Allometric scaling assist scientists to exchange doses between species during research, experiments, and clinical trials.
- Different equations described in this review could be used for dose extrapolation among species.
- Allometric scaling is generally used to convert doses among the species and is not preferred within species.

Synopsis:

1. Enlist the vehicles used in pharmacological experiments with concentrations.
2. Describe the calculation used for converting human to animal dose.

Experiment No. 02
Antiallergic Activity by Mast Cell Stabilization Assay

Aim: *To determine antiallergic activity by mast cell stabilization assay.*

Principle:

Mast cells are one of the major effector cells in the immune response system. Activated mast cells release pro-inflammatory cytokines, such as tumor necrosis factor (TNF)-α, interleukin (IL)-6, IL-8, IL-13 and inflammatory mediators, including histamine, luekotrienes, serotonin, prostaglandin (PG)E_2, as well as PGD_2). Cytokines, such as TNF-α, IL-6 and IL-8, are released in a co-ordinated fashion and play important roles in chronic inflammation. TNF-α is either preformed and stored in granules of mast cells, or is newly synthesized following mast cell activation; it is a multifunctional cytokine and an important mediator of the immune and inflammatory response. In contrast, IL-8 from mast cells act on surrounding cells such as neutrophils, T-lymphocytes and eosinophils, and plays a role in the activation of inflammatory effector cells. Calcium (Ca^{2+}) acts as a second messenger during cell activation, and an increase in intracellular Ca^{2+} concentration has been proposed as an essential trigger for mast cell activation.

Requirement:

Animal: Rat/mice (200 g/20 g).

Chemicals: 0.9% w/v NaCl, compound 48/80, Toluidine Blue, 2% gluteraldehyde solution, 0.2 M Sodium Phosphate buffer.

Method:

(i) *In-vitro* Passive Mast Cell Degranulation:

The sera of the active anaphylaxis induced animals to be collected and used for the passive mast cell degranulation. Briefly, 0.05 mL of serum to be incubated with equal volume of antigen (Horse serum and triple antigen), normal rat serum and peritoneal mast cell suspension from a donor rat for 3 min at 37°C in an eppendorf tube. The mixture to be incubated for 3 min and to be mixed with freshly prepared 2% gluteraldehyde solution in 0.2 M Sodium Phosphate buffer. The cell mixtures to be subjected for centrifuged 300 rpm for 15 min at 4°C. The cellular pellets obtained to be resuspended in a minimum amount of supernatant solution and the supernatant to be discarded. A smear is to be prepared on slide by taking 0.05 mL of the suspension. The smear to be allowed for drying and then stained with 0.1% toluidine blue and mast cells to be counted. Results are to be expressed as the percentage of degranulated and intact mast cells.

(ii) *In-vivo* Mast Cell Degranulation in Mice :

Three days after drug treatment schedule has to be followed. On day fourth each mice will be injected with 4 ml/kg, 0.9% w/v NaCl solution into peritoneal cavity. By gentle massage, peritoneal fluid will be collected after 5 min and transfer into siliconised test tube containing 7-10 RPMI-1640 buffer medium (pH 7.2 - 7.4). The content in test tubes has to be centrifuged at 400-500 rpm for 2-3 minutes. Pellet of mast cell has to be washed with same buffer medium twice by centrifugation, discarding supernatant. The cells will be challenged with **compound 48/80** (50 µg) and incubated at 37 °C in a water-bath for 10 min. Followed by staining with 1% toluidine blue, the cells has to be observed under microscope (45 X). Total 100 cells has to be counted from different visual area. Percentage protection against degranulation has to be calculated.

Sr. No.	Treatment Group	Dose mg/kg p.o.	No. of mast cell degranulated per cubic mm	% Protection of mast cell degranulation
1.	Control			-
2.	Standard			

Report:

Synopsis:
1. Explain the principle involved in hypersensitivity.
2. Enlist the **pro-inflammatory mediators.**

Experiment No. 03
Study of Anti-Ulcer Activity of a Drug Using Pyloric Ligation [Shay] Rat Model

Aim: *To study Anti-Ulcer Activity of a Drug Using Pyloric Ligation Shay Rat Model.*

Principle:

Gastric juice is digestive fluid composed of hydrochloric acid which digests proteins by activating digestive enzymes. The gastric mucosal lining is coupled with feedback systems to regulate its secretion. The gastrin hormone secreted by G cells in gastric antrum act on entero chromaffin-like cells in the gastric corpus to release histamine. Histamine via H_2-receptors stimulates the parietal cells to secrete gastric acid in to lumen of stomach.

The cause of gastric ulcers is *H. pylori*, NSAIDS, Crohn's disease, hypergastriaemia, hyperthyroidism and ulcerogenic agents like indomethacin, aspirin, reserpine. Besides gastric ulcers can be produced by hypothermic restraint stress and by pyloric ligation rat technique which is a valuable method to evaluate anti-ulcer activity.

Requirements:

Animals: Wistar rats (150-170g); Standard drug: Ranitidine 15 mg/kg; Saline-0.1N NaOH; Scissors, Suturing needle, Thread, cork board; Centrifugation tubes.

Procedure:

- Female Wistar rats weighing 150–170 g to be starved for 24 hours but having access to drinking water ad *libitum*.

- During this time, they are to be housed single in cages with raised bottoms of wide wire mesh in order to avoid cannibalism and coprophagy.

- Ten animals to be used per dose and as controls. Under ether anesthesia a midline abdominal incision has to be made.

- The pylorus to be ligated, care has to be exercised that neither damage to the blood supply nor traction on the pylorus.

- Grasping the stomach with instruments is to be meticulously avoided; else ulceration will invariably develop at such points.

- The abdominal wall to be closed by sutures. The test compounds to be given either orally by gavage or injected subcutaneously.

- The animals have to be placed for 19 hours in plastic cylinders with an inner diameter of 45 mm being closed on both ends by wire mesh.

- Afterwards, the animals to be sacrificed under CO_2 anesthesia.

- The abdomen to be opened and a ligature to be placed around the esophagus close to the diaphragm.

- The stomach has to be removed, and the contents are to be drained into a centrifuge tube.
- Along the greater curvature the stomach has to be opened and pinned on a cork plate.
- The mucosa to be examined with help of a stereomicroscope. In the rat, the upper two fifths of the stomach form the rumen with squamous epithelium and possess little protective mechanisms against the corrosive action of gastric juice.
- Below a limiting ridge, in the glandular portion of the stomach, the protective mechanisms are better in the mucosa of the medium two fifths of the stomach than in the lowest part, forming the antrum. Therefore, lesions occur mainly in the lumen and in the antrum.
- The number of ulcers to be noted and the severity to be recorded with the following scores:
  - ➢ 0 = no ulcer
  - ➢ 1 = superficial ulcers
  - ➢ 2 = deep ulcers
  - ➢ 3 = perforation
- The volume of the gastric content to be measured. After centrifugation, acidity is determined by titration with 0.1 N NaOH.

Ulcer Score	Observations
0	No ulcer
1	Superficial ulcer
2	Deep ulcer
3	Perforation

Evaluation:

$$\textbf{Ulcerative Index: (UI)} = \frac{UN + US + UP}{10}$$

Where, UN = Average number of ulcer per animal; US = Average severity scores; UP = Percentage of animals with ulcer.

Formula for Calculating % Ulcer Protection:

$$\% \text{ Ulcer Protection} = \frac{\text{Ulcer index in control} - \text{Ulcer index in test}}{\text{Ulcer index in control}} \times 100$$

For Acidity:

$$\text{Acidity} = \frac{\text{Volume of NaOH} \times \text{Normality} \times 100}{0.1} \times m.\ Eq/l/100\ g$$

Observations:

Group	Body Weight	Dose (mg/kg)	Volume (ml)	pH	Acidity (mEq/l/100 g)		Gastric erosion				Ulcer Index	% Ulcer Protection
							Ulcer score					
					Free	Total	0	1	2	3		

Report:

Synopsis:

1. Explain pathophysiology of peptic ulcer.

Experiment No. 04
Study of Anti-Ulcer Activity of Drug by NSAIDs

Aim: *To study Anti-Ulcer Activity of a Drug by NSAIDs (Indomethacin) Induced in Rat Model.*

Principle:

Non-steroidal anti-inflammatory drugs (NSAIDs) such as indomethacin, aspirin and ibuprofen are known to cause gastric ulcers, especially when abused. This model is important in investigating the potential usefulness of anti-secretory and cytoprotective agents since the underlying pathophysiology involves gastric acid secretion and mucosal prostaglandin synthesis. It is the most commonly used ulcer model in antiulcer studies. The frequency of usage could be attributed to the fact that NSAID induced peptic ulcers are the second most common etiology of peptic ulcers aside those caused by *Helicobaceter pylori*. NSAIDs are known to induce ulcers by inhibiting prostaglandin synthetase in the cyclooxygenase pathway. Prostaglandins are found in many tissues including the stomach, where they play a vital protective role via stimulating the secretion of bicarbonate and mucus, maintaining mucosal blood flow and regulating mucosal cell turnover and repair. Thus, the suppression of prostaglandin synthesis by NSAIDs results in increased susceptibility to mucosal injury and subsequently gastric ulceration.

Requirements:

Animals: Wistar rats (150-170 g); Drugs: omeprazole 20 mg/kg, indomethacin 100 mg/kg; Saline: 0.1N NaOH; Scissors, Cork board.

Procedure:

- Female Wistar rats weighing 150 – 170 g to be starved for 48 hours having access to drinking water ad libitum and divided into three groups (n = 6).
- Normal control, ulcer control (indomethacin group, 100 mg/kg), (omeprazole group, n = 30).
- Each group to be dosed with saline (control group) and omeprazole (Standard group) orally daily for 10 consecutive days before induction of ulcer by indomethacin.
- Indomethacin (ulcer inducing) to be given as a single oral dose (100 mg/kg). Four hours later after indomethacin treatment, the rats to be sacrificed and gastric tissue to be obtained for calculation of **Ulcer Index (U.I.)**.

Quantification of Ulceration:

- Cleaned stomachs will be pinned on a corkboard and ulcers will be scored using dissecting microscope with square-grid eyepiece based on grading on a '0' to '5' scale (depicting severity of vascular congestions and lesions/hemorrhagic erosions) as presented in observational table.
- Areas of mucosal damage to be expressed as a percentage of the total surface area of the glandular stomach estimated in square milli meters.

- Mean ulcer score for each animal to be expressed as ulcer index (U.I.) and the percentage of inhibition against ulceration to be determined by using the expressions:

$$\textbf{U.I.} = \left[\frac{\text{Ulcerated area}}{\text{Total stomach area}}\right] \times 100.$$

% Ulcer inhibition = [U.I. in control − U.I. in test] × 100/U.I. in control.

Ulcer Scores and Descriptive Remark:

Ulcer Score	Observations
0	Almost normal mucosa
1	Vascular congestions
2	One or two lesions
3	Severe lesions
4	Very severe lesions
5	Mucosa full of lesions

Observations:

Group	Body Weight	Dose(mg/kg)	Gastric erosion						Ulcer Index	% Ulcer Protection
			Ulcer score							
			0	1	2	3	4	5		

Report:

Synopsis:

1. Discuss the principle involved in NSAIDs induced gastric ulcer.
2. Enlist various drugs inducing gastric ulcer.

✍ ✍ ✍

Experiment No. 05
Study of Effect of Drugs on Gastrointestinal Motility

Aim: *To Determine the Drug Effect on Gastrointestinal Motility in Rat/Guinea pig/Rabbit.*

Introduction:

Intestinal motility is regulated by the enteric nervous system of the gut and the activity of this system can be modified by autonomic nervous system. Hence, effect of sympathomimetic and parasympathomimetic drugs on intestinal motility can be studied by using isolated piece of intestine. Parasympathomimetic drugs stimulate enteric neurons to release acetylcholine at neuromuscular junctions and enhance muscle tone and rhythmicity of intestine. Sympathomimetic drugs acts on α and β receptors and releases adrenaline which in turn prevents release of acetylcholine and inhibits muscle tone and rhythmicity. Animal models can be employed to study intestinal motility of sympathomimetic and parasympathomimetic drugs. Guinea pig ileum is advantageous for assay purposes as it produces steady baseline for studying effects of drugs. Rabbit intestine (ileum, deuodenum, jejunum) usually jejunum is used for the effects of pendular movements (continuous contraction and relaxation.

Requirements:

Animal: Rat (200 g)/ Guinea pig (300 – 350 g, over night fasted)/ Rabbit (1.5 kg)

Drug: Agonist : Acetylcholine

        Antagonist : Atropine

Apparatus: Organ bath thermostatically controlled, Kymograph, fulcrum, frontal writing lever, reservoir etc.

Physiological solution: Tyrode solution

Experimental Conditions:

Temperature	–	37°C
Bath volume	–	15 mL
Time cycle	–	3 min (30 sec-base line, 30 sec – response, 2 min – washing)
Tension of lever	–	1 g
Magnification	–	1 : 9
Aeration	–	Atmospheric air

Procedure:

- An adult rabbit/rat 1.5 kg/200 g to be head-blow and exsanguinate.
- Cut open the abdomen with a sharp scissor and remove the jejunum along with the mesentery.
- Keep it moist by Tyrode solution during further dissection.
- Spread out the jejunal loop and its mesentery to visualize the blood vessel in it. Adrenergic fibres run along with these vessels.
- Select a segment of jejunum along with it accompanying section of mesentery and place on a shallow dish containing Tyrode's solution.

- Tie a fine thread to the apex of the mesentery and place over a bipolar stimulating electrode. Connect this electrode to square wave pulse generator. Tie one end of the jejunum to oxygenating tube in the bath and the other to the Starling lever.
- Fill the bath with Tyrode solution maintained at 37°C.
- Electrical stimulation of the mesentery leads to stimulation of sympathetic nerve fibres, which produces inhibition of the pendular movements. It is necessary to allow longer time for relaxation (3 min).
- Use carbogen [Oxygen (95%) and carbon dioxide (5%)] for aeration rather than air.
- Electrical stimulation to be given at the rate of 50 shocks/sec of 10 volts strength for 30 sec duration. Elicit control responses to electrical stimulation and then add adrenaline and record its effect on these responses. Now add the test drug to the bath fluid and again elicit responses to electrical stimulation with adrenaline.
- Adrenergic neuron blocker inhibits responses to electrical stimulation but does not modify responses to both electrical stimulation and adrenaline.

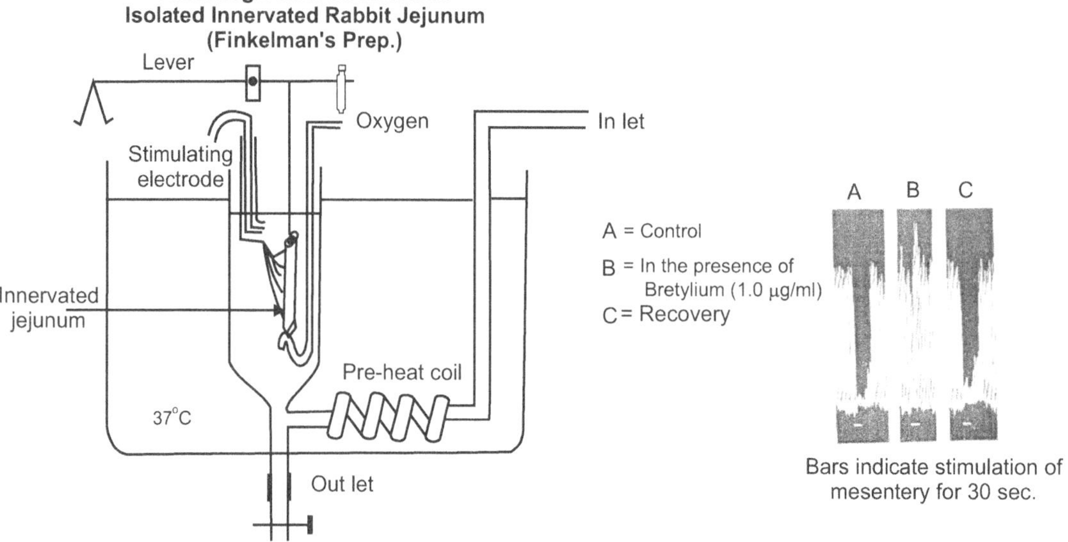

Fig. 1

(i) Apparatus showing the organ bath with stimulator connected to the mesentery.

(ii) Demonstration of site of action of AD neuron blocker.

Report:

Synopsis:

1. Describe the principle involved in Intestinal motility regulated by the enteric nervous system.

Experiment No. 06
Effect of Agonist and Antagonist Using Isolated Guinea Pig Ileum

Aim: *To determine the agonistic and antagonistic effect of the given drugs using isolated guinea pig ileum.*

Principle:

The effect of agonist and antagonist on isolated ileum will be first described by Magnus. This method is used to study the spontaneous contractions of the longitudinal and circular musculature and the inhibiting effect of atropine. And also used to study the effects of adrenaline on the lower segments causing contraction and on the segments of the upper end causing relaxation or to study the origin of acetylcholine release from guinea-pig intestine and longitudinal muscle strips retaining or being denervated from Auerbach's plexus responsible for generating peristaltic movement. This method is used as a basic screening model for determination of spasmolytic activity using ileum, duodenum and colon, whereby an anti-acetylcholine/anti carbachol property indicate anti-muscarinic activity and an anti-$BaCl_2$- property indicate musculo tropic, papaverine-like effect.

Requirements:

Animal: Guinea pig (300 – 350 g, over night fasted)

Drug: Agonist : Acetylcholine

Antagonist : Atropine

Apparatus: Organ bath thermostatically controlled, Kymograph, fulcrum, frontal writing lever, reservoir etc.

Physiological solution: Tyrode solution

Experimental Conditions:

Temperature   –   37°C

Bath volume   –   15 mL

Time cycle   –   3 min (30 sec-base line, 30 sec – response, 2 min – washing)

Tension of lever   –   1 g

Magnification   –   1 : 9

Aeration   –   Atmospheric air

The agonists and antagonists are as follows:

Sr. No	Agonist	Antagonist
1.	Acetylcholine 10–7 g/ml	Scopolamine 10–8–10–9 g/ml; Atropine 10–8–19–9 g/ml
2.	Carbachol 10–7 g/ml	Atropine 10–8–10–9 g/ml
3.	Histamine 10–6 g/ml	Histamine antagonists
4.	$BaCl_2$ 10–4 g/ml	Papaverine 10–5–10–6 g/ml
5.	Serotonin 10–6 g/ml	Serotonin antagonists
6.	PGE_2 2×10^{-7} g/ml	PG-antagonists

Procedure:

1. Cut open the abdomen and lift the caecum to trace the ileo-caecal junction. Cut and remove a few centimeters long of the ileal portion and immediately place it in the watch glass containing tyrode solution. Trim the mesentery and with gentle care clean the contents of the ileum by pushing the tyrode solution in to the lumen of the ileum. Utmost care should be taken to avoid any damage to the gut muscle. Cut the ileum in to small segments of 2-3 cm long.

2. Take one piece of ileum of 2-3 cm long and tie the thread to top and to the bottom ends without closing the lumen, and mount the tissue in the organ bath containing tyrode solution maintained at 35°C and bubbled with oxygen or air. A tension of 0.5 g is applied and the tissue is allowed to equilibrate for 30 min before adding drug to the organ bath.

3. Record concentration dependent responses due to acetylcholine using frontal writing lever. Contact of 30 sec and 3 min time cycles are followed for proper recording of the responses.

4. Record at least six responses due to increasing doses of acetylcholine or till you get the maximum response. The maximum response is achieved if one gets same or slightly less response with a higher concentration.

5. Then add the potential antagonist 5 min before the concentration-response curve is reobtained.

6. Properly label the graph and fix the tracing with the help of fixing solution.

7. Measure the height of the response in terms of mm.

Note: The obtained values can also be used to calculate the molar and log-molar concentrations (X-axis) and plot the graph against percentage response curves (Y-axis) of acetylcholine. Then determine the potency of antagonist of acetylcholine by calculating the PD2 value (which is defined as negative logarithm of the molar concentration of an antagonist that causes a 50% reduction of agonist's maximal response).

Agonistic and antagonistic effect of the given drugs using
isolated guinea pig ileum (Agonist-ACh; Antagonist -Atropine)

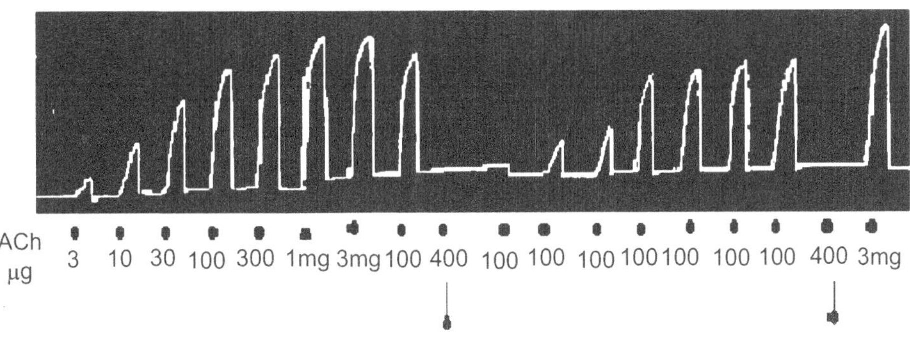

Fig. 1

Observations:

Sr. No.	Conc. of ACh (μ g/ml)	ACh concentration		Dose response in absence of atropine		Dose response in presence of atropine	
		µg/ml	Log Conc.	Response (mm)	% Response	Response (mm)	% Response
1.							
2.							
3.							
4.							
5.							

Report:

Synopsis:

1. Define agonist and antagonists with examples.
2. Describe the principle involved in agonist and antagonist effect on guinea pig ileum.

☙ ☙ ☙

Experiment No. 07
Estimation of Serum Biochemical Parameters by Using Semi Auto-Analyzer/Colorimeter

Aim (A): *To estimate the amount of serum alanine amino transferase (ALT or SGOT) present in the given blood sample.*

Reagents:

1. Substrate: Dissolve 5 g alanine and 20 mg α ketoglutaric acid in about 30 ml phosphate buffer and adjust the pH to 7.4 with 10% NaOH and then make up to 100 ml with phosphate buffer. Preserve with a few drops of chloroform in the cold.
2. Standard pyruvate: Dissolve 22 mg pyruvate in 100 ml phosphate buffer.
3. Phosphate buffer pH 7.4: Dissolve 68 g KH_2PO_4 in about 200 ml of water. Adjust pH 7.4 with 10% NaOH and make up to 500 ml.
4. 2,4-dinitrophenylhydrazine (DNPH): Dissolve 200 mg of 2,4-dinitrophenyl hydrazine in hot 1N HCl and make up to 1 liter with the acid.
5. 0.4 N NaOH (16 g/l).
6. Aniline citrate: Dissolve 50 g citric acid in 50 ml water, to this add an equal volume of redistilled aniline and mix.

Principle:

In the estimation of ALT (SGPT), serum is treated with alanine and ketoglutarate which are used as substrate. The new keto acid formed in the reaction namely pyruvate is treated with 2,4-diinitrophenylhydrazine. The absorbance of resultant brown color due to 2,4-initrophenylhydrazone is measured under alkaline conditions at 520 nm.

Procedure:

Take four test tubes. Mark them **T** for Test, **C** for Control, **S** for Standard and **B** for Blank and proceed as under:

Reagent (ml)	Blank	Standard	Test	Control
1. Buffered substrate	1.0	0.9	1.0	1.0
2. Serum	–	–	0.2	–
3. Standard	–	0.1	–	–
4. Water	0.2	–	–	–
5. Buffer	–	0.2	–	–
Incubate at 37°C for 30 minutes				
Aniline citrate	–	–	1 drop	1 drop
Serum	–	–	–	0.2
DNPH	1.0	1.0	1.0	1.0
Mix and allow to stand for 20 minutes at room Temperature				
0.4 N NaOH	10.0	10.0	10.0	10.0

Mix well, and take the reading in Photometer at 520 nm.

Calculation:

$$\text{ALT (SGPT)} = \left(\frac{AT - AC}{AS}\right) \times 16 \text{ I.U./L.}$$

Interfering substances:

Drug and toxic substances, which are detoxified by the liver cells, can result in elevated level of this enzyme. Paracetamol overdose and steroids in contraceptive pills have been reported to elevate the enzyme level.

Hemolysed sample should be avoided, as RBCs are rich in these enzymes.

Interpretation:

- Normal serum level of ALT (SGPT) ranges 5-40 I.U./L.
- It is known that liver is the richest source of ALT.
- ALT level is expected to increase during liver damage.
- ALT level also increases in heart disease but very small increase is observed as compared to ALT.

Liver diseases:

- **Infective hepatitis:** ALT increase, an increase begins in prodromal period when the determination can be of great value in testing suspected cases of infective hepatitis.
- **Jaundice:** Activity is maximal in two early stages of jaundice, then falling if recovery takes place.
- **Cirrhosis:** Elevation of enzymes is upto 5 times.
- **Hepatic Tumors:** Primary and secondary hepatic tumors cause an elevation of both enzymes with ALT higher than ALT.

Report:

The amount of ALT (SGPT) present in the given blood sample is ________ I.U./L.

✐ ✐ ✐

Aim (B): *To estimate the amount of serum glutamate pyruvate Transaminse (AST or SGPT) present in the given blood sample.*

Reagents:

1. Substrate: Dissolve 5 g alanine and 20 mg α-ketoglutaric acid in about 30 ml phosphate buffer and adjust the pH to 7.4 with 10% NaOH and then make upto 100 ml with phosphate buffer. Preserve with a few drops of chloroform in the cold.
2. Standard pyruvate: Dissolve 22 mg pyruvate in 100 ml phosphate buffer.
3. Phosphate buffer pH 7.4: Dissolve 68 g KH_2PO_4 in about 200 ml of water. Adjust pH 7.4 with 10% NaOH and make up to 500 ml.
4. 2,4-dinitrophenylhydrazine (DNPH): Dissolve 200 mg of 2,4-dinitrophenylhydrazine in hot 1N HCl and make up to 1 liter with the acid.
5. 0.4 N NaOH (16 g/l).
6. Aniline citrate: Dissolve 50 g citric acid in 50 ml water and to this add an equal volume of redistilled aniline. Mix.

Principle:

In the estimation of AST, serum is treated with alanine and α-ketoglutarate which are used as substrate. The new keto acid formed in the reaction namely pyruvate is treated with 2,4-dinitrophenylhydrazine. The absorbance of resultant brown color due to 2,4-dinitrophenylhydrazone is measured under alkaline conditions at 520 nm.

Procedure:

Take four test tubes. Mark them **T** for Test, **C** for Control, **S** for Standard and **B** for Blank and proceed as under:

Reagent (ml)	Blank	Standard	Test	Control
1. Buffered substrate	1.0	0.9	1.0	1.0
2. Serum	–	–	0.2	–
3. Standard	–	0.1	–	–
4. Water	0.2	–	–	–
5. Buffer	–	0.2	–	–
Incubate at 37°C for 30 minutes				
Aniline citrate	–	–	1 drop	1 drop
Serum	–	–	–	0.2
DNPH	1.0	1.0	1.0	1.0
Mix and allow to stand for 20 minutes at room temperature.				
0.4 N NaOH	10.0	10.0	10.0	10.0

Mix well, and take the reading in Photometer at 520 nm.

Calculation:

$$\text{AST or SGOT} = \left(\frac{AT - AC}{AS}\right) \times 16 \text{ I.U./L}$$

Interfering Substances:

Drug and toxic substances, which are detoxified by the liver cells, can result in elevated level of this enzyme. Paracetamol overdose, steroids in contraceptive pills have been reported to elevate the enzyme level.

Hemolysed sample should be avoided, as RBCs are rich in these enzymes.

Interpretation:

- Normal serum level AST or SGOT ranges 5-40 I.U./L.
- It is known that liver is the richest source of AST.
- AST level is expected to increase during liver damage.
- AST level also increases in heart disease but very small increase is observed as compared to AST.

Liver Diseases:

- **Infective hepatitis:** AST increase, an increase begins in prodromal period when the determination can be of great value in testing suspected cases of infective hepatitis.
- **Jaundice:** Activity is maximal in two early stages of jaundice, then falling if recovery takes place.
- **Cirrhosis:** Elevation of enzymes is up to 5 times.
- **Hepatic Tumors:** Primary and secondary hepatic tumors cause an elevation of both enzymes with AST higher than ALT.

Report:

The amount of AST or SGPT present in the given blood sample is _________ I.U./L.

Synopsis:

1. Describe the principle involved in estimation of SGOT/SGPT.
2. Explain the significance and importance of SGOT/SGPT with normal range.

✍ ✍ ✍

Experiment No. 08
Effect of Saline Purgative on Frog Intestine

Aim: *To evaluate effect of saline purgative on frog/rat intestine.*

Introduction:

Laxatives are used in the treatment of constipation to promote the emptying of feces. Laxatives produce their effect by several mechanisms. The four main types of laxatives include: saline purgatives, fecal softeners, contact purgatives and bulk laxatives. Saline purgatives are the salts and contain highly charged ions that do not readily cross biological membrane, therefore remain inside the lumen or passageway of the bowel.

By retaining water through osmotic forces, saline purgatives increase the volume of the contents of the bowel, stretching the colon and producing a normal stimulus for contraction of the muscle which leads to defecation. Some commonly used salts are magnesium sulphate, magnesium hydroxide, sodium sulphate and potassium sodium tartrate.

Requirements:

Animals: Frog/Rat.

Reagents: 0.9 to 0.45% of saline (hypotonic), 27% magnesium sulphate (hypertonic), Frogs Ringer solution (isotonic).

Instruments: Cork board, pithing needle, dissecting instruments, needle with thread, tuberculin syringe with needle.

Procedure:

- Pith the frog/ decapitate rat and place it on a dissecting board.
- Expose the abdominal cavity and carefully trace the small intestine.
- Make the small intestine into three compartments by tying threads of different colours in such a way that no fluid can move from one compartment to other.
- Inject 0.2 ml of each hypotonic solution into first compartment, 0.2 ml of hypertonic solution to second compartment and 0.2 ml of isotonic solution into third compartment.
- Wait for 20 min and the observations are to be recorded.

Observation:

Drug	Compartment	Effect
Hypotonic solution (0.2 ml of 0.9% of saline)	First	Shrunken
Hypertonic solution (0.2 ml of 27% magnesium sulphate)	Second	Swollen
Isotonic solution (0.2 ml of frog`s Ringer solution)	Third	No change

Conclusion:

- Hypotonic solution causes the fluid to move from lumen into circulation by the process of osmosis which leads to shrinks the tissue.
- Hypertonic solution which moves the fluid from cell into the lumen and cause swelling the tissue.
- Where isotonic solution did not shows any movement of the fluid across the intestinal membrane.

Report:

Synopsis:

1. Describe isotonic, hypertonic and hypotonic solutions and its importance.

🖋 🖋 🖋

Experiment No. 09
Insulin Hypoglycemic Effect in Rabbit

Aim: *To evaluate the effect of insulin in rabbits at different intervals.*

Introduction:

Insulin is a peptide hormone produced by the β cells of pancreas in response to high glucose level in the blood. A released insulin act on the insulin receptors on body cells and activates glucose transporters to absorb more glucose into the cells thereby regulates carbohydrates, protein and fat metabolism in body cells. Reduced blood glucose levels inhibits insulin release and stimulates α-cells of pancreas to release glucagon to maintain glucose levels in the blood by glycogenolysis and gluconeogenesis.

The aim of the experiment is to evaluate the effect of insulin in rabbits at different intervals.

Requirements:

Animals: Rabbits weighing 1.8-2.2 kg.

Drugs: 20 units of insulin preparation.

Reagents: Normal saline, HCl, 0.5% Phenol, 1.4 - 1.8% glycerin.

Procedure:

- Select healthy rabbits weighing 1.8-3.2 kg for the study.
- The animals should be maintained in uniform diet for 7 days.
- The animals to be fasted for 18 hours with no access to water before starting the procedure.
- Select three animals for the study and inject 1 unit/ml of insulin.
- Prepare the drug solution freshly before administration.
- Weigh 20 units of insulin accurately and dissolve in normal saline.
- Acidify the solution by using concentrated HCl and adjust pH 2.5.
- Add 0.5% of phenol as a preservative and 1.4-1.8% of glycerin and make the final volume to 20 units/ml of solution.
- Withdraw 2 ml of blood from marginal ear vein of each rabbit and estimate blood glucose level by using suitable method.
- The concentration of glucose can be noted down as initial blood glucose level.
- Then inject insulin (1 unit/ml) to the animals and check the blood sugar level up to 5 hours at the interval of 1 hour each.
- Determine blood glucose levels as final blood sugar levels and compare both initial and final blood glucose levels.

Observations:

Sr. No.	Initial blood glucose level (mg/ml)	Final glucose level at Different time intervals in (hour)			
		1	2	3	4
1.					
2.					
3.					
Average					

Conclusion:

Mean percentage decrease of blood glucose levels at different time intervals which determine the effects of insulin.

Report:

Synopsis:

1. Enlist insulin preparations.
2. Describe the role of insulin in management of diabetes.

Experiment No. 10
Test for Pyrogen (Rabbit Method)

Aim: *To evaluate pyrogen test for given sample using rabbit.*

Introduction:

The pyrogen test is aim to check the existence of pyrogen by using rabbits. The pyrogen test is based on the measurement of the increase in the rabbit's temperature upon being injected with a product that might contain a contaminant of the pyrogen type. The pyrogen, as their name suggests, refer to all the substances that cause an increase in fever, also known as pyrexia. Upon entering into contact with pyrogens, rabbits have an increase in their temperature, just like humans. For this reason and since they are animals used in laboratories for different purposes, they are chosen to conduct this test.

Test Animals:

Use healthy mature rabbits each weighing not less than 1.5 kg which have not lost body mass when kept on a constant diet for not less than one week. Do not use the rabbits repeatedly in the same test unless as long a resting period as possible is taken. Animals should be excluded which have been used for a previous test that will be decided as pyrogen positive.

Record the rectal temperature 4 times at 2 hours intervals during 1 to 3 days prior to the test. House the animals individually during this period in an area free from disturbances likely to excite them, and exercise particular care to avoid disturbances on the day of the test.

Keep the temperature in an area of performing test uniform between 20°C and 27°C and preferably maintain constant humidity for at least 48 hours before the test.

Apparatus:
1. **Thermometer:** Use a rectal thermometer or any other temperature recording devices of equal sensitivity for which the time necessary for reading the rectal temperature is known.
2. **Syringe and injection needle:** Render the syringes and needles Pyrogen free by heating at 250°C for not less than 30 minutes.

Test Procedure:
*   Quantity of injection: Unless otherwise specified, 10 mL of the sample per kg of body mass of the animals is used/injected.
*   Perform the test at an environmental temperature similar to that of the room where in the animals are housed.
*   The test animals are usually fixed in a suitable type of holder (rabbit holder).
*   Insert the rectal thermometer or other temperature recording device into the rectum of the test animal to a constant depth in the range of 60 to 90 mm, and read the temperature after a sufficient period of time.

- Withhold food from the test animals beginning several hours before the first temperature recording and until the test is completed.
- Determine the temperature of the test animals three times at 1 hour intervals before the injection of the sample.
- When the second and third temperatures show little difference, the latter is taken as the control temperature.
- Do not use animals whose second and third temperatures are not in accord or exceed 39.8°C even if these two values are similar.
- Warm the sample to 37°C before injection, and administer intravenously through an ear vein within 15 minutes after the third temperature recording.
- Hypotonic solution other than Water for Injection may be made isotonic by the addition of pyrogen free sodium chloride before the test.
- Read the temperatures three times at 1 hour intervals after injection.
- The difference between the control temperature and the highest temperature is taken to be the rise in body temperature.

Interpretation of results:

- The test is carried out on a group of three rabbits. If 2 or 3 rabbits show an individual rise of 0.6°C or more above the respective control temperature, the test shall be considered as positive.
- If only one animal shows a temperaturer is of 0.6°C or more, or if the sum of the temperature rises of the three animals exceeds 1.4°C, repeat the test on a group of five other rabbits.
- The test will be considered positive, if two or more of the five rabbits show an individual temperature rise of 0.6°C or more.
- When the Pyrogen test is positive, the sample is considered to be rejected.

Disadvantages/Limitations:

- It is a long test and therefore, the temperature of the animal needs to be measured during the 3 hours following the injection, at approximately 30-minute intervals.
- If it is thought that many other substances which are both endogenous and exogenous could be causing the increase in the rabbit's temperature.
- It is an inadequate method to determine pyrogens in medicines, such as steroids etc.
- A very important disadvantage is the fact that the content of endotoxins that are present in a sample cannot be quantified by this test, which only offers a qualitative result.

Report:

Synopsis:

1. Describe the principle involved in Pyrogen test.

✍ ✍ ✍

Experiment No. 11
Determination of Acute Oral Toxicity (LD$_{50}$) of a Drug from a Given Data

Aim: *To determine the acute oral toxicity (LD$_{50}$) of the drug from given data.*

Principle:

The principle involved in acute oral toxicity studies is that, based on a step-wise method with the use of the least number of animals per stage, adequate information is acquired on the acute toxicity of the substance to facilitate its classification. The test substance is administered orally to a group of experimental animals at one of the defined doses. The substance is tested employing a step-wise procedure, each step using three animals of a single-sex (normally females). Absence or presence of compound-related mortality of the animals treated at one step can verify the consequent step, that is;

- No further testing is needed,
- Dosing of three further animals, with the same dose
- Dosing of three further animals at consequent higher or consequent lower dose level.

The method will enable a judgment with respect to classifying the test substance to one of a series of toxicity classes defined by fixed LD50 cut-off values.

Requirements:

Animal: Rat (Ideally), other rodent species may be used.

Sex: Females (nulliparous and non-pregnant)

Age: 8 to 12 weeks old

Dose: 1 mL/100 g of body weight

Procedure:

- Animals to be fasted prior to dosing (with the rat, food however not water ought to be withheld over-night, with the mouse, food however not water ought to be withheld for 3-4 hours).
- Test substance to be administered in a single dose by gavage using a stomach tube or an appropriate intubation cannula.
- After the administration of test substance, food may be withdrawn for another 3-4 hours in rats or 1-2 hours in mice.
- Three animals are used for each step. The selected dose level starting from 1 of 4 fixed levels, 5, 50, 300 and 2000 mg/kg of body weight. The initial dose level should be that which is most likely to produce mortality in some of the dosed animals.
- A limit test at a dose level of 2000 mg/kg body weight will be performed with six animals (three animals per step). Remarkably, a limit test at a dose level of 5000 mg/kg will be performed with three animals.
- If test substance-related mortality is occurred, further examining will be done for the next lower level.

- Animals will be observed individually after dosing during the first thirty minutes, occasionally during the first 24 hours, with special consideration given during the first 4 hours, and daily subsequently, for a total of 14 days.

- Observations will be done to assess if the animals continue to display signs of toxicity which include changes in skin and fur, eyes and mucous membranes, and also respiratory, circulatory, autonomic nervous systems and central nervous systems, and somatomotor activity and behaviour pattern. Additionally observations to be made for occurrence of tremors, convulsions, salivation, diarrhoea, lethargy, sleep and coma.

Observation:

Table 1: Determination of LD_{50}

Group	Dose (mg/kg)	Log dose	% Dead	*Corrected %	Probits
1	25	1.4	0	2.5	**3.04**
2	50	1.7	40	40	**4.75**
3	75	1.88	70	70	**5.52**
4	100	2	90	90	**6.28**
5	150	2.18	100	97.5	**6.96**

*Corrected % Formula for 0 and 100 is given in the text.

Table 2: Transformation of percentage mortalities to probits

%	0	1	2	3	4	5	6	7	8	9
0	–	2.67	2.95	3.12	3.25	3.36	3.45	3.52	3.59	3.66
10	3.72	3.77	3.82	3.87	3.92	3.96	4.01	4.05	4.08	4.12
20	4.16	4.19	4.23	4.26	4.29	4.33	4.36	4.39	4.42	4.45
30	4.48	4.50	4.53	4.56	4.59	4.61	4.64	4.67	4.69	4.72
40	4.75	4.77	4.80	4.82	4.85	4.87	4.90	4.92	4.95	4.97
50	5.00	5.03	5.05	5.08	5.10	5.13	5.15	5.18	5.20	5.23
60	5.25	5.28	5.31	5.33	5.36	5.39	5.41	5.44	5.47	5.50
70	5.52	5.55	5.58	5.61	5.64	5.67	5.71	5.74	5.77	5.81
80	5.84	5.88	5.92	5.95	5.99	6.04	6.08	6.13	6.18	6.23
90	6.28	6.34	6.41	6.48	6.55	6.64	6.75	6.88	7.05	7.33

Report:

Synopsis:

1. Describe the process involved in LD_{50} determination.

Experiment No. 12
Determination of Acute Skin Irritation/Corrosion of a Test Substance

Aim: *To determine the acute skin irritation/corrosion of a test substance.*

Principle:

The test substance should be applied in a single dose on the skin of the experimental animal. The untreated skin areas of the test animal serve as the control. The extent of irritation/corrosion is read and scored at particular intervals and is further described to provide a complete evaluation of the effects. The duration of the study should be adequate to evaluate the reversibility or irreversibility of the effects observed.

Animals showing long-lasting signs of severe distress and/or pain at any phase of the test should be humanely killed, and the substance is evaluated accordingly.

Requirements:

Animals: Albino rabbit.

Dose level: 0.5 ml of liquid or 0.5 g of solid or paste.

Procedure:

- The initial test should be performed using one animal, especially when the substance is suspected to have corrosion potential.

- The test substance should be applied to a small area (approximately 6 cm^2) of skin and covered with a gauze patch, which is held in place with non-irritating tape. In case if the direct application is not possible (e.g., liquids or some pastes), the test substance should first be applied to the gauze patch, which is then applied to the skin.

- At the end of the exposure phase, which is usually 4 hours, remaining test substance should be removed using water or an appropriate solvent without altering the existing response.

- All animals should be observed for signs of erythema and oedema, and the reactions will be scored at sixty minutes, and then at 24, 48 and 72 hours after removal of the patch. For the initial test, the site of the test is also observed immediately after the patch has been removed.

- If there is any damage to the skin which cannot be recognized as irritation or corrosion at 72 hours, observations may be required until day 14 to conclude the reversibility of the effects.

- Additionally, toxic effects like defatting of the skin, and any general adverse effects (e.g., effects on clinical signs of toxicity and body weight) ought to be fully depicted and recorded. The histopathological examination should be considered to elucidate equivocal responses.

- If no corrosive effect is observed in the initial test, the irritant or negative response should be confirmed using two additional animals, each with one patch, for an exposure phase of 4 hours. If an irritant effect is seen in the initial test, the confirmatory test may be conducted in a sequential manner, or by exposing two additional animals simultaneously.

SCORE OF SKIN REACTIONS

Erythema and Eschar Formation:

No erythema - 0

Very slight erythema (barely perceptible) - 1

Well defined erythema - 2

Moderate to severe erythema - 3

Severe erythema (beef redness) to eschar formation preventing grading of erythema - 4

Oedema Formation:

No oedema - 0

Very slight oedema (barely perceptible) - 1

Slight oedema (edges of area well defined by definite raising) - 2

Moderate oedema (raised approximately 1 mm) - 3

Severe oedema (raised more than 1 mm and extending beyond area of exposure) - 4

Observation:

	Score of Skin Reactions	
	Erythema and Eschar Formation	**Oedema Formation**
Initial Test		
1		
Confirmatory Test		
2		
3		
Mean		

Report:

Synopsis:

1. Describe the principle involved in skin irritation as per OECD guidelines.

Experiment No. 13
Determination of Acute Eye Irritation/Corrosion of a Test Substance

Aim: *To determine the acute eye irritation/corrosion of the test substance.*

Principle:

The substance to be tested is applied in a single dose to one of the eyes of the experimental animal, following pretreatment with a systemic analgesic and induction of appropriate topical anaesthesia; the untreated eye serves as the control. The extent of eye irritation/corrosion is evaluated by scoring lesions of conjunctiva, cornea, and iris, at specific intervals. Other effects within the eye and adverse general effects are delineating to produce a whole analysis of the effects. The duration of the study should be sufficient to evaluate the reversibility or irreversibility of the effects.

Animals showing signs of severe distress and/or pain at any stage of the test or lesions consistent with the humane endpoints should be humanely killed, and the substance assessed accordingly.

Requirements:

Animal: Albino rabbit

Dose levels: For liquids – 0.1 ml of test substance

For solids – < 100 mg of test substance

Procedure:

- Buprenorphine 0.01 mg/kg to be administered by subcutaneous injection (SC) 60 minutes prior to test substance to provide a therapeutic level of systemic analgesia.

- One or two drops of a topical ocular anaesthetic (e.g. 0.5% proparacaine hydrochloride or 0.5% tetracaine hydrochloride) to be applied to each eye 5 minutes before administration of test substance.

- The test substance ought to be placed within the conjunctival sac of one eye of each animal once gently propulsion the lower lid off from the eyeball.

- The lids are then gently held together for about one second in order to prevent loss of the material.

- The other untreated eye will to be served as control.

- Buprenorphine 0.01 mg/kg SC and meloxicam 0.5 mg/kg SC are to be administered after 8 hours of the test substance to provide a continued therapeutic level of systemic analgesia.

- After the first 8 hours of test substance treatment, buprenorphine 0.01 mg/kg SC should be administered every 12 hours, in conjunction with meloxicam 0.5 mg/kg SC every 24 hours, until the ocular lesions resolve and no clinical signs of pain and distress are present.

- Observations should be performed and recorded at a minimum of 1 hour, 24 hours, 48 hours, 72 hours, 7 days, 14 days, and 21 days in order to determine the status of the lesions, and their reversibility or irreversibility. The grades of ocular lesions should be recorded at each examination. Any other lesions in the eye (e.g. pannus, staining, anterior chamber changes) or adverse systemic effects should also be reported.

- Reactions to be examined by using a binocular loupe, hand slit-lamp, biomicroscope, or other suitable devices.

- After recording the observations at twenty-four hours, the eyes could also be examined with the help of fluorescent dye.

GRADING OF OCULAR LESIONS

Cornea:

No ulceration or opacity – 0

Scattered or diffuse areas of opacity; details of iris clearly visible – 1

Easily discernible translucent area; details of iris slightly obscured – 2

Nacrous area; no details of iris visible; size of pupil barely discernible – 3

Opaque cornea; iris not discernible through the opacity – 4

Iris:

Normal – 0

Markedly deepened rugae, congestion, swelling, moderate circumcorneal hyperaemia; or injection; iris reactive to light -1

Hemorrhage, gross destruction, or no reaction to light – 2

Conjuctivae:

Normal – 0

Some blood vessels hyperaemic – 1

Diffuse, crimson colour; individual vessels not easily discernible – 2

Diffuse beefy red – 3

Chemosis:

Normal – 0

Some swelling above normal – 1

Obvious swelling, with partial eversion of lids – 2

Swelling, with lids about half closed – 3

Swelling, with lids more than half closed – 4

Observation:

Sr. No.	GRADING OF OCULAR LESIONS			
	Cornea	Iris	Conjunctivae	Chemosis
1.				
2.				
3.				
4.				
5.				
6.				
Mean				

Report:

Synopsis:

1. Describe the principle involved in eye irritation as per OECD guidelines.

Experiment No. 14
Calculation of Pharmacokinetic Parameters from a given Data

Aim: *To calculate pharmacokinetic Area Under the Curve (AUC) parameters from the given data.*

Background:

Area under the curve (AUC) represents area under the 'plasma concentration versus time curve'. It is the total integrated area under the plasma level time curve and expressed in total amount of drug that comes into the systemic circulation followed by its administration. AUC is expressed in µg/ml.hr. It is the most important parameter in evaluating the bioavailability of a drug from the dosage form as it represents the extent of absorption.

Trapezoidal rule method: In this method, plasma concentration versus time plot used for the determination of AUC is divided into geometric figures whose area can be determined individually using the appropriate geometric formula for each figure. Therefore, the plasma concentration versus time plot is drawn with straight lines. Thus, when two adjacent concentration points are joined with a straight line, and perpendicular on the X-axis is drawn from this two concentration points, one obtains a geometric figure. With the exception one or two segments, all segments in this plot tend to be trapezoids, hence the name trapezoidal rule.

Area of triangle = (1/2) (height) (base)

Area of trapezoid = (1/2) (the sum of the two parallel sides) (base)

AUC by

Trapezoidal = 1 $[(C_1 + C_2) (t_2 - t_1) + (C_2 + C_3) (t_3 - t_2) + \dots + (C_{n-1} + C_n) (t_n - t_{n-1})]$

Method:

Calculation of AUC Using the Trapezoidal Rule

Time (hr)	0	1	2	3	4	5	6
Concentration (µg/ml)	100	50	25	12.5	6.25	3.13	1.56

AUC for the first time interval:

$$AUC_1 = \frac{C_0 + C_1}{2} \times time_{(1 - 0)}$$

$$AUC_1 = \frac{100 + 50}{2} \times 1 \text{ hr} = 75 \text{ µg.hr/ml}$$

AUC for the second time interval:

$$AUC_2 = \frac{C_1 + C_2}{2} \times time_{(2 - 1)}$$

$$AUC_2 = \frac{50 + 25}{2} \times 1 \text{ hr} = 37.5 \text{ µg.hr/ml}$$

Similarly calculate the AUC_3, AUC_4, AUC_5 and AUC_6

Therefore, $AUC_{(c_0 - c_6)} = [(AUC_1) + (AUC_2) + (AUC_3) + (AUC_4) + (AUC_5) + (AUC_6)]$

$AUC_{(c_0 - c_6)} = 147.657$ µg.hr/ml

Observations:

Time (hr)	Concentration (µg/ml)	time interval (hr)	AUC	Area (µg.hr/L)
0	100	–	–	–
1	50	1	75	75
2	25	1	37.5	112.5
3	12.5	1	18.75	131.25
4	6.25	1	9.375	140.625
5	3.13	1	4.688	145.313
6	1.56	1	2.344	147.657
			***AUC (c_0 – c_6) =**	**147.657**

*AUC_{0-t} last

Report: Area under curve for the given plasma-time profile is **147.657** µg. hr/ml.

Synopsis:

1.   Define AUC, $T_{1/2}$ and C_{max}.

Experiment No. 15
Biostatics Methods in Experimental Pharmacology

Aim: *Biostatistics methods in experimental pharmacology.*

Introduction:

Statistics is a way of thinking about variable data. Statistics implies both, data and statistical methods. It can be considered as an art as well as science. Statistics can neither prove nor disprove anything. Statistics may be defined as the method concerned with the handling of numerical data derived from a group of individuals. These individuals may be either humans, animals or other organisms. Biostatistics is a branch of statistics employed to biological or medical sciences. Biostatistics comprises the contributions and applications of health, medicines and nutrition with other fields such as biology, epidemiology and genetics. The statistical method has two major branches mainly descriptive and inferential. Descriptive statistics explain the distribution of population measurements by providing types of data, estimates of central tendency (mean, mode and median), and measures of variability (standard deviation, correlation coefficient), whereas inferential statistics are used to express the level of certainty about estimates and includes hypothesis testing, standard error of mean, and confidence interval.

Types of Data:

Observations recorded during research constitute data. There are three types of data i.e. nominal, ordinal, and interval data. Statistical methods for analysis mainly depend on the type of data. Generally, data show a picture of the variability and central tendency. Therefore, it is very important to understand the types of data

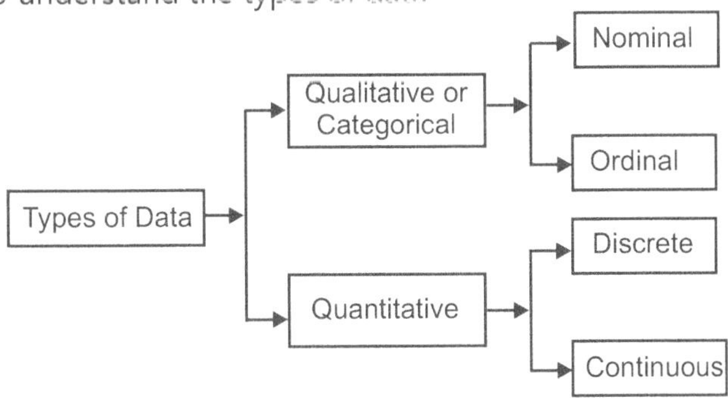

Fig. 1

1. Nominal data: This is similar to categorical data where data is simply selected "names" or categories based on the presence or absence of some characteristics/attributes without any ranking between the categories. For example, patients are categorized by gender as males or females; by religion like Hindu, Muslim, or Christian. It also includes binominal data, which refers to two possible outcomes. For example, the outcome of cancer may be death or survival, drug therapy with drug 'X' will show improvement or no improvement at all.

2. Ordinal data: It is also called as ordered, categorical, or graded data. Generally, this type of data is expressed as scores or ranks. There is a common order between categories, and they can be arranged or ranked in order. For example, pain may be categorised as mild, moderate and severe. Considering there is a method between the three grades of pain, this type of data is called as ordinal. To indicate the intensity of pain, it may also be expressed as scores (mild = 1, moderate = 2, severe = 3). Hence, data can be arranged in an order and rank.

3. Interval data: This type of data is characterized by an equal and definite interval between two measurements. For example, weight is denoted as 20, 21, 22, 23, 24 kg. The interval between 20 and 21 is the same as that between 23 and 24. Interval type of data can be either continuous or discrete. A continuous variable can select any value within a given range. For example, haemoglobin (Hb) level may be taken as 11.3, 12.6, 13.4 g % while a discrete variable is usually assigned integer values i.e. does not have fractional values. For example, blood pressure values are generally discrete variables or the number of cigarettes smoked per day by a person. Sometimes, certain data may be converted from one form to another form to reduce skewness and make it follow the normal distribution. For example, drug doses are converted to their log values and plotted in a dose-response curve to obtain a straight line so that analysis becomes easy.

Measures of Central Tendencies:

Mean, median and mode are the three measures of central tendencies.

Mean is the general measure of fundamental tendency, most extensively used in calculations of averages. It is least affected by sampling fluctuations. The mean of several individual values (X) is always nearer the true value of the individual value itself. Mean exhibits less variation than that of individual values, therefore they provide confidence in applying them.

Median is an average, which is obtained by getting middle values of a set of data arranged or ordered from lowest to the highest (or vice versa). In this process, 50% of the population has the value smaller than and 50% of samples have the value larger than the median. It is used for scores and ranks. Median is a more reliable indicator of primary value when one or more of the lowest or highest observations are wide distant or are not evenly distributed. Median in case of even number of observations is considered randomly as an average of two middle values, and in case of an odd number, the primary value determines the median.

Mode is the most common value, or it is the point of maximum concentration. Most fashionable number, which occurred repeatedly, contributes mode in the distribution of quantitative data. The mode is used when the values are widely varying and is rarely used in medical studies. For skewed distribution or samples where there is wide variation, mode and median are useful.

Problem 1:

Find the mean of the following data set: 56, 35, 45, 67, 12, 24, 48, 55, 58, 30.

Solution: 56 + 35 + 45 + 67 + 12 + 24 + 48 + 55 + 58 = 430/10 = 430/10 = 43.

The mean = 43.

The median is the number in an ordered set of data that is in the middle.

If we have a set of data with an odd number of data points then the median is the data point in the middle.

1, 2, 3, <u>4</u>, 5, 6, 7

If we have a set of data with an even number of data points, then the median is the mean of the two data points in the middle

1, 2, 3, <u>4</u>, <u>5</u>, 6, 7, 8

4 + 5/2 = 9/2 = 4.5

The mode is the most common number in the set of data.

Mode = 4.5.

Standard Deviation:

In addition to the mean, the degree of variability of responses has to be indicated since the same mean may be obtained from different sets of values. Standard deviation (SD) explains the variability of the observation of the mean.

To describe the scatter of the population, the most useful measure of variability is SD.

Correlation Coefficient: Correlation is a relationship between two variables. It is used to measure the degree of a linear relationship between two continuous variables. It is represented by 'r'. In the Chi-square test, we do not get the degree of association, but we can know whether they are dependent or independent of each other. Correlation may be due to any direct relationship between two variables. This also may be due to a few inherent factors common to both variables. The correlation is expressed in terms of the coefficient. The correlation coefficient values are constantly between −1 and +1. If the variables are not correlated, then the correlation coefficient is zero. The maximum value of 1 is obtained if there is a straight line in the scatter plot and considered as a perfect positive correlation. The association is positive if the values of x-axis and y-axis tend to be high or low together. On the contrary, the association is negative i.e. −1 if the high y-axis values tend to go with low values of the x-axis and considered as a perfect negative correlation. Larger the correlation coefficient, stronger is the association. A weak correlation may be statistically significant if the numbers of observation are large. Correlation between the two variables does not necessarily suggest the cause and effect relationship. It indicates the strength of association for any data in comparable terms as, the correlation between height and weight, age and height, weight loss and poverty, parity and birth weight, socioeconomic status and haemoglobin. While performing these tests, it requires x and y variables to be normally distributed. It is generally used to form a hypothesis and to suggest areas of future research.

Problem 2:

The following data points represent the weight (in kilograms) of each of Newman's four dogs.

6, 2, 3, 1

Solution: Step 1: Find out mean : (6 + 2 + 3 + 1 = 12/4) = 3

Step 2: Find out variance: $\sqrt{\dfrac{14}{4}} = \sqrt{3.5} = 1.87$

Step 3: SD = 1.87

Types of Distribution:

Though this universe is full of uncertainty and variability, a large set of experimental/biological observations always tend towards a normal distribution. This unique behaviour of data is the key to entire inferential statistics. There are two types of distribution.

1. Gaussian/normal distribution: If data is symmetrically distributed on both sides of mean and form a bell-shaped curve in frequency distribution plot, the distribution of data is called normal or Gaussian. The noted statistician professor Gauss developed this, and therefore, it was named after him. The normal curve describes the ideal distribution of continuous values i.e. heart rate, blood glucose level and Haemoglobin %. Whether our data is normally distributed or not, can be checked by putting our raw data of study directly into computer software and applying distribution test. Statistical treatment of data can generate some useful measurements, the most important of which are mean and standard deviation of the mean. In an ideal Gaussian distribution, the values present between the points 1 SD below and 1 SD above the mean value (i.e. ± 1 SD) will hold 68.27% of all values. An ideal distribution of the values; the mean, mode, and median are equal within-population under study. Even if distribution in the original population is far from normal, the distribution of sample averages tends to become normal as the size of the sample increases. This is the single most important reason for the curve of normal distribution. Various methods of analysis are available to make assumptions about normality, including 't' test and analysis of variance (ANOVA). In a normal distribution, skew is zero. If the difference (mean - median) is positive, the curve is positively skewed and if it is (mean - median) negative, the curve is negatively skewed, and therefore, the measure of central tendency differs.

2. Non-Gaussian (non-normal) distribution: If the data is skewed on one side, then the distribution is non-normal. It may be binominal distribution or Poisson distribution. In binominal distribution, the event can have only one of two possible outcomes such as yes/no, positive/negative, survival/death, and smokers/non-smokers. When the distribution of data is non-Gaussian, different test like Wilcoxon, Mann-Whitney, Kruskal-Wallis, and Friedman test can be applied depending on the nature of data.

Standard Error of Mean:

This is the estimated standard deviation for the distribution of sample means for an infinite population. It is the sample standard deviation divided by the square root of sample size, n.

Applications of Standard Error of Mean:

1. To determine whether a sample is drawn from the same population or not when its mean is known.
2. To work out the limits of desired confidence within which the population mean should lie. For example, take fasting blood sugar of 200 lawyers. Suppose mean is 90 mg% and SD = 8 mg%. With 95% confidence limits, fasting blood sugar of lawyer's would be; n = 200, SD = 8; hence $\text{SEM} = \dfrac{SD}{\sqrt{n}} = \dfrac{8}{\sqrt{200}} = \dfrac{8}{14.14} = 0.56$. Hence,

   Mean fasting blood sugar + 2 SEM = 90 + (2 × 0.56) = 91.12 while

   Mean fasting blood sugar − 2 SEM = 90 − (2 × 0.56) = 88.88

Therefore, confidence limits of fasting blood sugar of lawyer's population are 88.88 to 91.12 mg %. If the mean fasting blood sugar of another lawyer is 80, we can say that he is not from the same population.

Confidence Interval (CI) Or (Fiducial Limits):

Confidence limits are two extremes of a range within which 95% observations will present. These explain the limits in which 95% of the mean values if determined in related experiments are likely to fall. The value of 't' corresponding to a probability of 0.05 for the suitable degree of freedom is read from the table of distribution. By multiplying this value with the standard error, the 95% confidence limits for the mean are collected as per formula below.

   Lower confidence limit = mean − (t 0.05 × SEM)

   Upper confidence limit = mean + (t 0.05 × SEM)

If n > 30, the interval M ± 2(SEM) will include M with a probability of 95% and the interval M ± 2.8(SEM) will include M with the probability of 99%. These intervals are, consequently, called the 95% and 99% confidence intervals, sequentially. The major difference within the 'p' value and confidence interval is that the confidence interval signifies clinical significance, whereas 'p' value shows statistical significance. Therefore, in many clinical studies, the confidence interval is preferred instead of 'p' value, and some journals specifically ask for these values.

Many journals apply mean and SEM to explain variability in the sample. The SEM is a measure of precision for an estimated population mean, whereas SD is a measure of data variability around the mean of a sample of the population. Hence, SEM is not descriptive statistics and should not be used as such. Correct use of SEM would be only to indicate the precision of the estimated mean of the population.

Null Hypothesis:

The primary object of statistical analysis is to find out whether the effect produced by a compound under study is genuine and is not due to chance. Therefore, the analysis normally attaches a test of statistical significance. The first step in such a test is to state the null hypothesis. In null hypothesis (statistical hypothesis), we assume that there exist no differences between the two groups. The alternative hypothesis (research hypothesis) states that there is a difference between the two groups. For example, a new drug 'A' is claimed to have analgesic activity and we want to test it with the placebo. In this investigation, the null hypothesis would be 'drug 'A' is not better than the placebo.' An alternative hypothesis would be 'there is a difference between new drug 'A' and placebo.' When the null hypothesis is accepted, the difference between the two groups is not significant. It means, both samples were drawn from a single population, and the difference obtained between two groups was due to chance. If the alternative hypothesis is proved i.e. null hypothesis is rejected, then the difference between the two groups is statistically significant. A difference between drug 'A' and placebo group, which would have arisen by chance is less than five per cent of the cases, that is less than 1 in 20 times is considered as statistically significant ($P < 0.05$). In any experimental procedure, there is the possibility of occurring two errors.

1. **Type I Error (False positive):** This is also known as α error. It is the probability of finding a difference; when no such difference exists, which results in the acceptance of an inactive compound as an active compound. Such an error, which is not unusual, may be tolerated because, in subsequent trials, the compound will reveal itself as inactive and thus finally rejected. For example, we proved in our trial that new drug 'A' has an analgesic action and accepted as an analgesic. If we commit type I error in this experiment, then a subsequent trial on this compound will automatically reject our claim that drug 'A' is having analgesic action and later on drug 'A' will be thrown out of the market. Type I error is fixed in advance by choice of the level of significance employed in the test. It may be noted that type I error can be made small by changing the level of significance and by increasing the size of the sample.

2. **Type II Error (False negative):** This is also called as β error. It is the probability of inability to detect the difference when it exists, thus resulting in the rejection of an active compound as an inactive. This error is more serious than type I error because once we labelled the compound as inactive, there is a possibility that nobody will try it again. Thus, an active compound will be lost. This type of error can be minimized by taking a larger sample and by employing sufficient dose of the compound under trial. For example, we claim that drug 'A' is not having an analgesic activity after a suitable trial. Hence, drug 'A' will not be tried by any other researcher for its analgesic activity and thus drug 'A', in spite of having analgesic activity, will be lost just because of our type II error. Hence, the researcher should be very careful while reporting the type II error.

Level of Significance:

If the **probability (P)** of an event or outcome is high, we assume it is not rare or not uncommon. But, if the P is low, we assume it is rare or uncommon. In biostatistics, a rare event or outcome is called significant, whereas a non-rare event is called non-significant. The 'P' value at which we regard an event or outcomes as enough to be regarded as significant is called the significance level. In research, generally P value less than 0.05 or 5% is considered as a significant level. However, on justifiable grounds, we may adopt a different standard like $P < 0.01$ or 1%. Whenever possible, it is better to give actual P values instead of $P < 0.05$. Even if we have found the true value or population value from the sample, we cannot be confident as we are dealing with a part of population only; howsoever big the sample may be. We would be wrong in 5% cases only if we place the population value within 95% confidence limits. Significant or insignificant indicates whether a value is likely or unlikely to occur by chance. 'P' indicates the probability of relative frequency of occurrence of the difference by chance.

Outliers:

Sometimes, when we examine the data, one value is very extreme from another value. Such value is indicated as outliers. This could be due to two reasons. Firstly, the value obtained may be due to chance; in that case, we should keep that value in the final analysis as the value is from the same distribution. Secondly, it may be due to mistake. Causes may be listed as typographical or measurement errors. In such cases, these values should be eliminated, to avoid invalid results.

One-tailed and Two-tailed Test:

When distinguishing two groups of continuous data, the null hypothesis is that there is no real difference within the groups (A and B). The alternative hypothesis is that there is a real difference between the groups. This difference could be in either direction e.g. A > B or A < B. When there is some assured way to understand in advance that the difference could only be in one direction e.g. A > B and when a good ground considers only one possibility, the test is called one-tailed test. Whenever we contemplate both the possibilities, the test of significance is known as a two-tailed test. For example, when we know that English boys are taller than Indian boys, the result will lie at one end that is one tail distribution; hence the one-tail test is used. When we are not sure of the direction of difference, it is always better to use a two-tailed test. For example, a new drug 'X' is supposed to have an antihypertensive activity, and we want to compare it with atenolol. In this case, as we don't know the exact direction of the effect of drug 'X', so one should prefer the two-tailed test. When you want to know the action of a particular drug is different from that of another, but the direction is not specific, always use a two-tailed test. At present, most of the journals use two-sided P values as a standard norm in biomedical research.

Importance of Sample Size Determination:

The sample is a fraction of the universe. Studying the universe is the best parameter. But, when it is possible to achieve the same result by taking a fraction of the universe, a sample is taken. Applying this, we are saving time, manpower, cost, and at the same time, increasing efficiency. Hence, adequate sample size is of prime importance in biomedical studies. If the sample size is too small, it will not give us valid results, and validity in such a case is questionable, and therefore, the whole study will be a waste. Furthermore, large sample requires more cost and manpower. It is a misuse of money to enroll more subjects than required. A good small sample is much better than a bad large sample. Hence, the appropriate sample size will be ethical to produce precise results.

Factors Influencing Sample Size Include:

1. Prevalence of particular event or characteristics: If the ubiquity is high, a small sample can be taken and vice versa. If ubiquity is not known, then it can be obtained by a pilot study.

2. Probability level considered for accuracy of the estimate: If we need more safeguard about conclusions on data, we need a larger sample. Hence, the size of the sample would be larger when the safeguard is 99% than when it is only 95%. If barely a small difference is suspected and if we need to identify even that small difference, then we need a large sample.

3. Availability of money, material, and manpower.

4. Time-bound study reduces the sample size as routinely observed with dissertation work in postgraduate courses.

Sample Size Determination and Variance Estimate:

To calculate sample size, the formula requires the knowledge of standard deviation or variance, but the population variance is unknown. Therefore, the standard deviation has to be estimated.

Frequently used sources for estimation of standard deviation are:

1. A pilot or preliminary sample may be drawn from the population, and the variance computed from the sample may be used as an estimate of standard deviation. Observations used in the pilot sample may be counted as a part of the final sample.

2. Estimates of standard deviation may be accessible from the previous or similar studies, but sometimes, they may not be correct.

Calculation of Sample Size:

Calculation of sample size plays a pivotal role while doing any research. Before the calculation of the sample size, the following five points are to be considered very carefully. First of all, we have to assess the minimum expected difference between the groups. Then, we have to find out the standard deviation of variables. Different methods for the determination of standard deviation have already been discussed previously. Instantly, set the level of significance (alpha level, generally set at $P < 0.05$) and Power of study (1-beta = 80%). After choosing all the parameters, we have to decide the formula from computer programs to take the sample size. We will operate on two examples to understand sample size calculation.

1. The mean (SD) diastolic blood pressure of hypertensive patient after enalapril therapy is found to be 88. It is claimed that telmisartan is better than enalapril, and a trial is to be conducted to find out the truth. By our convenience, suppose we take the minimum expected the difference between the two groups is 6 at the significance level of 0.05 with 80% power. Results will be analyzed by unpaired 't' test. In this case, the minimum expected difference is 6, SD is 8 from the previous study, the alpha level is 0.05, and power of the study is 80%. After putting all these values in the computer program, sample size comes out to be 29. If we take allowance to non-compliance and dropout to be 4, the final sample size for each group would be 33.

2.   The mean haemoglobin (SD) of the newborn is observed to be 10.5 (1.4) in the pregnant mother of the low socioeconomic group. It was decided to carry out a study to decide whether iron and folic acid supplementation would increase the haemoglobin level of the newborn. There will be two groups, one with supplementation and other without supplementation. Minimum difference expected between the two groups is taken as 1.0 with 0.05 level of significance and power as 90%. In this example, SD is 1.4 with a minimum difference of 1.0. After keeping these values in the computer-based formula, sample size comes out to be 42 and with an allowance of 10%, the final sample size would be 46 in each group.

How to Choose an Appropriate Statistical Test?

There are many tests in biostatistics, but selection mainly depends on characteristics and type of analysis of data. Sometimes, we necessitate to find out the variance between means or medians or association between the variables. The number of groups used in a study may vary; therefore, study design also varies. Hence, in such a situation, we will have to make a decision which is more precise while selecting the appropriate test. The inappropriate test will lead to invalid conclusions. Statistical tests can be divided into parametric and non-parametric tests. If variables follow the normal distribution, data can be subjected to the parametric test, and for non-Gaussian distribution, we should apply a non-parametric test. The statistical test should be decided at the start of the study. Following are the different parametric test used in the analysis of various types of data.

1.   Student's 't' Test:

Mr W. S. Gosset, a civil service statistician, introduced 't' distribution of small samples and published his work under the pseudonym 'Student.' This is one of the most widely used tests in pharmacological investigations, involving the use of small samples. The 't' test is always applied for analysis when the number of samples is 30 or less. It is normally applicable for graded data like blood glucose level, body weight, height etc. If the sample size is more than 30, 'Z' test is applied. There are two types of 't' test, paired and unpaired.

When to apply paired and unpaired:

1.   When comparison has to be made between two measurements in the same subjects after two consecutive treatments, paired 't' test is used. For example, when we want to compare the effect of drug A (i.e. decrease blood sugar) before the start of treatment (baseline) and after 1 month of treatment with drug A.

2.   When a comparison is made between two measurements in two different groups, the unpaired 't' test is used. For example, when we analyse the effects of drug A and drug B (i.e. mean change in blood glucose level) after one month from baseline in both groups, unpaired 't' test' is applicable.

Examples:

(i) Calculate a paired t test by hand for the following data:

Sr. No.	Score 1	Score 2
1	3	20
2	3	13
3	3	13
4	12	20
5	15	29
6	16	32
7	17	23
8	19	20
9	23	25
10	24	15
11	32	30

Solution:

Step-1: Subtract each Y score from each X score.

Step-2: Add up all of the values from Step 1. Set this number aside for a moment.

Step-3: Square the differences from Step 1.

Step-4: Add up all of the squared differences from Step 3.

Step-5: Use the formula to calculate the t-score.

Sr. No.	Score 1	Score 2	X − Y	$(X - Y)^2$
1	3	20	−17	289
2	3	13	−10	100
3	3	13	−10	100
4	12	20	−8	64
5	15	29	−14	196
6	16	32	−16	256
7	17	23	−6	34
8	19	20	−1	1
9	23	25	−2	4
10	24	15	9	81
11	32	30	2	4
SUM			**−73**	**1131**

$$t = \frac{(\Sigma D)/N}{\sqrt{\dfrac{\Sigma D^2 - \left(\dfrac{(\Sigma D)^2}{N}\right)}{(N-1)\,(N)}}}$$

$$t = \frac{-73/11}{\sqrt{\dfrac{1131 - \left(\dfrac{5329}{11}\right)}{110}}}$$

$$t = \frac{-73/11}{\sqrt{\dfrac{1131 - \left(\dfrac{(-73)^2}{11}\right)}{(11-1)\,(11)}}} \qquad t = -2.74$$

Step 6: Find the p-value in the t-table, using the degrees of freedom. If you do not have a specified alpha level, use 0.05 (5%).

For this sample problem, with df = 10, **the t-value is 2.228**.

Step 7: Compare your t-table value from Step 6 (**2.228**) to your calculated t-value (−2.74). The calculated t-value is greater than the table value at an alpha level of 0.05. *The p-value is less than the alpha level: p <0.05.*

(2) ANOVA:

When we need to compare two sets of unpaired or paired data, the student's 't' test is implemented. Yet, when there are three or more sets of data to examine, we want the help of well-designed and multi-talented method called as an analysis of variance (ANOVA). This test compares multiple groups at one time. In ANOVA, we draw the assumption that each sample is randomly drawn from the normal population, and also they have the same variance as that of population. There are two types of ANOVA.

1. One way ANOVA:

It compares three or more unmatched groups when the data are categorized in one way. For example, we may analyse a control group with three varying doses of aspirin in rats. Here, there are four unmatched groups of rats. Hence, we should apply one way ANOVA. We should take repeated measures ANOVA test when the trial uses matched subjects. For example, the effect of supplementation of vitamin C in each subject before, during, and after the treatment. Matching should not be based on the variable you are comparing. For example, if you are comparing blood pressures in two groups, it is better to match based on age or other variables, but it should not be to match based on blood pressure. The term repeated measures apply strictly when you give treatments repeatedly to one subjects. ANOVA works well even if the distribution is only approximately Gaussian. Therefore, these tests are used routinely in many fields of science. The P-value is calculated from the ANOVA table.

2. Two way ANOVA:

Also called two factors ANOVA, determines how a response is affected by two factors. For example, you might measure a response to three different drugs in both men and women. This is a complicated test. Therefore, we think that for postgraduates, this test may not be so useful.

Importance of post hoc test:

Post-tests are the modification of 't' test. They account for multiple comparisons, as well as for the fact that the comparison is interrelated. ANOVA only directs whether there is a significant difference between the various groups or not. If the results are significant, ANOVA does not tell us at what point the difference between various groups subsists. But, the post-test is capable to pinpoint the exact difference between the different groups of comparison. Therefore, post-tests are very useful as far as statistics are concerned. There are five types of post-hoc test namely; Dunnett's, Turkey, Newman-Keuls, Bonferroni, and test for linear trend between mean and column number.

Three sets of five mice are randomly selected to be placed in a standard maze but with different colour doors. The response is the time required to complete the maze as seen below. Perform the appropriate analysis to test if there is an effect due to door colour. (Use α = 0.01).

Colour	Time				
Red	9	11	10	9	15
Green	20	21	23	17	30
Black	6	5	8	14	7

Step 0 : Check Assumptions

Step 1 : Hypotheses

$$H_0 \; : \; \mu_{Red} = \mu_{Green} = \mu_{Black}$$
$$H_a \; : \; \text{at least one inequality}$$

Step 2 : Significance Level

$$\alpha \; = \; 0.01$$

Step 3 : Critical Value and Rejection Region

Critical Value: $F_{a, (df_1 = k - 1, df_2 = N - k)} = F_{0.01 (df_1 = 2 df_2 = 12)} = 6.93$

Reject the null hypothesis if $F \geq 6.93$.

Step 4 : Construct the One-way ANOVA Table

$$\sum_{i=1}^{k} \frac{(T_i)^2}{n_i} = \frac{(9 + 11 + 10 + 9 + 15)^2}{5} + \frac{(20 + 21 + 23 + 17 + 30)^2}{5} + \frac{(6 + 5 + 8 + 14 + 7)^2}{5}$$

$$= \frac{(54)^2}{5} + \frac{(111)^2}{5} + \frac{(40)^2}{5} = 3367.4$$

$$\frac{(T)^2}{N} = \frac{(9 + 11 + 10 + 9 + 15 + 20 + 21 + 23 + 17 + 30 + 6 + 5 + 8 + 14 + 7)^2}{15}$$

$$= \frac{(205)^2}{15} = 2801.6667$$

$$\sum_{i=1}^{k} \sum_{j=1}^{n_i} y_{ij}^2 = 9^2 + 11^2 + 10^2 + 9^2 + 15^2 + 20^2 + 21^2 + 23^2 + 17^2 + 30^2 + 6^2$$
$$+ 5^2 + 8^2 + 14^2 + 7^2$$
$$= 3537$$

$$\text{SSTr} = \sum_{i=1}^{k} \frac{(T_i)^2}{n_i} - \frac{(T)^2}{N} = 3367.4 - 2801.6667 = 565.7333$$

$$\text{SSE} = \sum_{i=1}^{k} \sum_{j=1}^{n_i} y_{ij}^2 - \sum_{i=1}^{k} \frac{(T_i)^2}{n_i} = 3537 - 3367.4 = 169.6$$

Source	df	SS	MS = SS/df	F-statistic	p-value
Treatments	2	565.7333	282.8667	20.0142	p-value < 0.001
Error	12	169.6000	14.1333		
Total	14	735.3333			

Step 5 : Decision – Since $20.0142 \geq 6.93$ (p-value ≤ 0.01), we shall reject the null hypothesis.

Step 6 : State conclusion in words – At the $\alpha = 0.01$ level of significance, there exists enough evidence to conclude that there is an effect due to door colour.

How to select a post test?
1. Select Dunnett's post-hoc test if one column represents the control group and we wish to compare all other columns to that control column but not to each other.
2. Select the test for linear trend if the columns are arranged in natural order (i.e. dose or time) and we want to test whether there is a trend so that values increases (or decreases) as you move from left to right across the columns.
3. Select Bonferroni, Turkey's, or Newman's test if we desire to compare all pairs of columns.

Following are the non-parametric tests used for the analysis of different types of data:

1. Chi-square test:

The Chi-square test is a non-parametric test of proportions. This test is not based on any assumption or distribution of any variable. This test, though different, follows a specific distribution known as Chi-square distribution, which is very useful in research. It is most commonly used when data are in frequencies such as the number of responses in two or more categories. This test involves the calculations of a quantity called Chi-square (x^2) from Greek letter 'Chi' (x) and pronounced as 'Kye.' It was developed by Karl Pearson.

Applications:
1. **Test of proportion:** This test is used to find the significance of the difference between two or more than two proportions.
2. **Test of association:** The test of association between two events in binomial or multinomial samples is the most important application of the test in statistical methods. It measures the probabilities of association between two discrete attributes. Two events can often be studied for their association such as smoking and cancer, treatment and outcome of disease, level of cholesterol and coronary heart disease. In these cases, there are two possibilities, either they influence or affect each other or they do not. In other words, you can say that they are dependent or independent of

each other. Thus, the test measures the probability (P) or relative frequency of association due to chance and also if two events are associated or dependent on each other. Varieties used are generally dichotomous e.g. improved / not improved. If data are not in that format, the investigator can transform data into dichotomous data by specifying above and below the limit. The multinomial sample is also useful to find out the association between two discrete attributes. For example, to test the association between numbers of cigarettes equal to 10, 11- 20, 21-30, and more than 30 smoked per day and the incidence of lung cancer. Since, the table presents the joint occurrence of two sets of events, the treatment and outcome of disease, it is called the contingency table (Con-together, tangle- to touch).

2. Wilcoxon-Matched-Pairs Signed-Ranks Test:

This is a non-parametric test. This test is used when data are not usually distributed in a paired design. It is also called as Wilcoxon-Matched Pair test. It analyses only the difference between the paired measurements for each subject. If the P-value is small, we can reject the idea that the difference is a coincidence and conclude that the populations have different medians.

3. Mann-Whitney test:

It is a Student's 't' test performed on ranks. For large numbers, it is almost as sensitive as Student's 't' test. For small numbers with unknown distribution, this test is more sensitive than Student's 't' test. This test is generally used when two unpaired groups are to be compared and the scale is ordinal (i.e. ranks and scores), which are not normally distributed.

4. Friedman test:

This is a non-parametric test, which compares three or more paired groups. In this, we have to rank the values in each row from low to high. The goal of using a matched test is to control experimental variability between subjects, thus increasing the power of the test.

5. Kruskal-Wallis test:

It is a non-parametric test, which compares three or more unpaired groups. Non-parametric tests are less powerful than parametric tests. Commonly, P values tend to be higher, executing it harder to identify real differences. Hence, firstly, try to transform the data. Sometimes, a trivial transformation will convert non-Gaussian data to a Gaussian distribution. The non-parametric test is considered only if the outcome variable is in rank or scale with only a few categories. In this case, the population is far from Gaussian or one or few values are off-scale, too high, or too low to measure.

✍ ✍ ✍

OUR UPCOMING BOOKS
As Per PCI Regulations Third Year (Semester VI)

- **Medicinal Chemistry III :** S.G. Walode
- **Medicinal Chemistry III :** K.G. Bothara
- **Practical Medicinal chemistry III :** S.G. Walode
- **Pharmacology III :** Dr. S. V. Tembhurne
- **Pharmacology III :** K.G. Bothara, K.K. Bothara
- **Practical Pharmacology III :** Dr. Arjun Patra
- **Herbal Drug Technology :** Vaibhav shinde, Ms. K. S. Bodas, S.B. Gokhale
- **Practical Herbal Drug Technology :** Vaibhav Shinde, Ms. K. S. Bodas, S.B. Gokhale
- **Biopharmaceutics and Pharmacokinetics :** Sunil bakliwal
- **Pharmaceutical Biotechnology :** Dr. Chandrakant Kokare
- **Medicinal Chemistry III :** Dr. Abhishek Tiwari
- **Pharmacology III :** Dr. Rupesh Gautam, Dr. Kalpesh Gour
- **Herbal Drug Technology :** Dr. Versha Tiwari, Dr. Vikash Sharma
- **Biopharmaceutics and Pharmacokinetics :** Hari Kumar
- **Pharmaceutical Biotechnology :** Dr. Khush Yadav, Mr. Rajiv Saxena, Ms. Satinder Kaur, Garima Joshi
- **Quality Assurance :** Bhupender Sing Tomar, Dr. Pawan Jhalwal, Surajpal verma
- **Medicinal Chemistry III :** Vibha Chandan Patil, Dr Chandrashekhar Narajji
- **Medicinal Chemistry III :** Mr. Mayur S. Jain, Mr. Mayur R. Bhurat, Sanjay A. Nagdev, Dr. Md. Rageeb Md. Usman
- **Practical Medicinal Chemistry III :** Dr. Sunita T. Patil, Dr. Md. Rageeb Md. Usman, Dr. Parloop A. Bhatt
- **Pharmacology III :** Dr. Manjunatha. P. Mudagal
- **Practical Pharmacology III :** Dr. Manjunatha. P. Mudagal
- **Herbal Drug Technology :** Kuntal Das
- **Herbal Drug Technology :** Dr. Santram Lodhi, Dr. Md. Rageeb Md. Usman, Dr. Tushar A. Deshmukh, Mr. Vaibhav M. Darvhekar
- **Practical Herbal Drug Technology :** Prof. Md. Rageeb Md. Usman, Prof. Vaibhav M. Darvhekar, Prof. (Dr.) Akhila S., Prof. (Dr.) Vijay Kumar D.
- **Biopharmaceutics and Pharmacokinetics :** Dr. B. Prakash Rao
- **Pharmaceutical Biotechnology :** Kuntal Das
- **A Practical Book Of Medicinal Chemistry (Combined Book Sem. IV & VI)**
  Dr. Abhishek Tiwari, Dr. Rajeev Kumar